MEDITATION WITH MARY JAYNE

How I Lost One Hundred Pounds with Marijuana Therapy

KEN KIZZEE

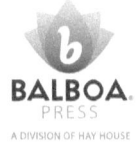

BALBOA
PRESS
A DIVISION OF HAY HOUSE

Balboa Press books may be ordered through booksellers or by contacting:

Balboa Press
A Division of Hay House
1663 Liberty Drive
Bloomington, IN 47403
www.balboapress.com
1-(877) 407-4847

Because of the dynamic nature of the Internet, any web addresses or links contained in this book may have changed since publication and may no longer be valid. The views expressed in this work are solely those of the author and do not necessarily reflect the views of the publisher, and the publisher hereby disclaims any responsibility for them.

The author of this book does not dispense medical advice or prescribe the use of any technique as a form of treatment for physical, emotional, or medical problems without the advice of a physician, either directly or indirectly. The intent of the author is only to offer information of a general nature to help you in your quest for emotional and spiritual well-being. In the event you use any of the information in this book for yourself, which is your constitutional right, the author and the publisher assume no responsibility for your actions.

Any people depicted in stock imagery provided by Thinkstock are models, and such images are being used for illustrative purposes only. Certain stock imagery © Thinkstock.

Printed in the United States of America.

ISBN: 978-1-4525-7747-0 (sc)
ISBN: 978-1-4525-7748-7 (e)

Library of Congress Control Number: 2013912168

Balboa Press rev. date: 7/2/2013

Table of Contents

INTRODUCTION

I was surrounded by love and miserable. I was unhealthy and the size of my waist told the world. A great and unique company that I was a part of was just purchased by a corporate vacuum cleaner.

Change was in the air; it was 2012 after all.

I of course had no idea what change was coming. As a matter of fact, I didn't even know who I was anymore. The world just wasn't making sense and I was starting to seriously worry if maybe, just perhaps, I may be losing my mind. I was horribly out of shape and thinking that this may be the beginning of an early end. My mind's incessant chatter was to the point of driving me crazy until, after one particularly bad day, I finally said to myself "I'm going to do whatever it takes to avoid being taken away in an ambulance."

Its 2013 now, my blood pressure is in check, my cholesterol is normal and I'm more than 100 pounds lighter. Weight really isn't as important as much as how I look and feel, and what I can now accomplish seemingly effortlessly. I do however, really feel great and look much slimmer. I'm constantly buying new, smaller clothes and I feel as if this is a permanent momentum. I use the word love more liberally in my everyday conversations and I'm off on an adventure that I had put off over twenty years ago. The concepts in this book aren't new and they are not mine; even if presumed to be original. This is the answer to that question that so many people around me have been asking. "How are you doing it?"

This short book is a story of awakening; finding myself and using that knowledge to change myself. It is not some secret recipe for brownies. It's a cumulative story-lesson that is best read through once in its entirety and then used as a reference. This story-lesson is how I went from unhealthy and negative to being relaxed and groovy in a very short amount of time with seemingly little to no effort; but with the assistance of marijuana therapy. Cannabis alone will not bring about change in your life. You have to set your intent; overcome your fears and declare that you will _____. Cannabis can help you to not only relax, but also to regain your balance, focus, and seemingly energize you; but only if you are open and aware enough to notice.

Fair warning, I am the son of a repressed hippy. Reader caution is advised.

I come from what I would think of as a normal New Jersey, middle class broken home. I couldn't wait to join the Army; and neither could my mother. I was the last of three children that she raised, but the only boy, and the last to leave the house. Having two older sisters, I was subject to all sorts of humiliation growing up that I'm sure in no way influences my homophobia; like being dressed up in a communion gown.

At seventeen, I had already held a job reliably for a couple of years and was promoted due to that (not a very high bar when working under the table). I was making good money for that age; I thought. I bought a Yugo on my own after all; but that's how we were raised. Hard working, reliable, always think of the other person first, humility, honor, integrity, loyalty, your place of work is like a temple you worship in every day; my Grandmother was fond of quoting that. Basically, you work within your means to do what you have to do. I really felt as if I was ready to tackle the world and I thought I had proven it to my mother. She let me enlist in the United States Army at the ripe old age of seventeen. I was to learn later however, from the time I started boot camp, she wouldn't leave the recruiter or the Army alone; acting like a drill sergeant herself. You see, if I didn't write home, my mother would worry and start calling people until she heard the answer she wanted; which was of course, that I would write a letter home periodically. I had been through basic and advanced training and was stationed in Germany when my commander summoned me to his office. He wasn't happy, as it appeared that he was under orders from HIS commander, to personally instruct me to write home.

My mother was of course a saint in my eyes but she was a New Yorker, a large woman in every aspect who knew how to throw her weight around when she needed to. If I can believe a childhood story, her dream was to run off to the Alps and become a nun like in The Sound of Music; she was very Catholic. The path she chose instead left her alone and broke, after having raised three children through some very rough times. I was the last child out of the house and I think the focus of her mental angst while she sat home alone in the dark. I believe she was a repressed hippy, always doing what she was supposed to do instead of doing what she wanted to do.

My mother died while I was in the service. She was obese. She had Phlebitis. The cause of death was a blood clot from her leg that clogged in her lung. She died in her sleep.

I remember my last days at home before joining the service. My mother appeared to be suffering from a condition but nobody knew what. In the evening, she would listen to music and spiritual teachings through headphones. She would cry for no apparent reason. She would nervously scratch her head to the point of creating a bald spot.

Flash forward twenty five years. At the office one day I suddenly had all the symptoms of a heart attack. I was in a meeting and my chest got tight, I started sweating, my arms went numb to my elbows. I stood to catch my breath but instead I lost it.

At 41 years old, roughly the same age that my mother was when I left for the service. I weighed in at 325 pounds and stood 5' 10" tall. I was a smoker. My blood pressure had the top of my head feeling like a percolating coffee pot, my cholesterol results were all the bad numbers; not enough of the good. My diet wasn't good either, but it wasn't all junk food; I was a typical meat and potatoes kind of guy. Very few people realized I was so out of shape because my frame carried it well but I knew; and I decided to seriously think about changing that. C'mon, you know what I mean. Let me hear from all of you fellow procrastinators who take just a big enough step in the right direction to plant a seed and then feel miserable for not following through. Drives me crazy too; or at least, it used to.

PRECIPICE

I had a successful career in information technology which all started because I like video games. When the personal computer arrived on the scene, my first was a Commodore 64. You could do some pretty amazing things for the time on it but you had to know how as some of the best video games required you to tweak or customize your computer if you wanted to play them. When I got out of the service, I found work servicing those computers for a private company to make their business applications work on them; that's all the opening it took for me. Despite my career, which is all I really focused on since leaving the Army, I had little else in my life. I had served in combat and saw not only death and destruction but great despair of those left alive as well. My grandparents and parents were both gone and my siblings and I just went our own separate ways early in life. I was never successful in love for long. I fail at life, or so I thought.

I was very good at one thing however; my chosen profession. Over the years, I punched my ticket in all the right places and went so far as to indebt myself with worldly goods to compensate for it. I had been in a couple of long term relationships but always found myself "wanting" more. My most recent relationship lasted around ten years, and included buying a house with a radiant woman whom I love to this day and thought I would eventually marry. What I now realize is that while our lives were compatible, our inner beings were not; more precisely, my inner being was nowhere to be found. As I now know, you have to find that before you can find yourself, and you need to find yourself before you can find another to share your life with. Marijuana therapy allowed me to relax and realize this.

The same underlying analytical principal was also true for overcoming my unhealthy physical situation. You have to find yourself and be able to understand your feelings and emotions before you can figure out how to fix yourself. All you really need to do is to listen to, and feel your "self" (emotions), listen to your body to understand what it's telling you and then learn how you can go about getting it done. Marijuana Therapy permitted me the clarity of higher thinking and focus in a peaceful state of mind, just long enough to figure this out. Sound like hippie nonsense?

Spirituality had eluded me since I was kicked out of catechism for asking too many questions. The priest had told my mother that I needed more faith in my life. I responded that I simply didn't believe what was being presented as it didn't make sense to me. My mother was wise enough to explain to me that I needed to find my own path. I was thirteen then and I think I get it now.

I use the phrase "inner being" sometimes to describe what my mother would refer to as the Holy Spirit; I think. What do I mean by inner being? Good question. The simple answer is this; whoever asked that question is who you are right now. You could be completely identified with or caught up in, your thoughts and emotions and that person could have asked the question. Or it could be the voice inside your head that asked you the question as you read it. You know the one I mean, the voice we sometimes hear and discount or shrug off altogether; regrettably so at times.

The voice inside your head that I'm referring to is the one that isn't associated with thought. That is your inner being-the nonjudgmental voice; the sound of peace, comfort and abundance. The one that makes you want to love and trust people, places and situations. The one that reminds you to accept life as it is, and that life only gives us what we need to grow. All we need to do is keep an eye out for it with an open mind as to grasp it.

At the office one day I suddenly had all the symptoms of a heart attack. I was in a meeting and my chest got tight, I started sweating, my arms went numb to my elbows. I stood to catch my breath but instead I lost it.

Excusing myself, I went to a friend, explained that I thought I was having a heart attack and asked him to drive me to the hospital. I believed what I said; I thought I was having a heart attack. When we got to the hospital, I walked into the emergency room and when asked, told the nurse I thought I was having a heart attack but then came my inner voice, in it's typical dry, drill sergeant tone; "sit down and relax; you're not going to die today".

The nurse put me in a cube, connected me to an EKG and did her thing, but all she could find was that an enzyme in my blood was elevated, which normally indicated a heart muscle injury. The doctors poked and prodded some more and wanted to admit me to the hospital for observation (or as malpractice insurance). I refused and asked my friend to assist in my escape… which we did, but only after I signed a statement refusing treatment; and then we went back to work. We were busy, you see. That's how we rationalized it in our heads as men but in truth, it was because we worked with a group of people who genuinely cared for one another and we knew we had to go back and tell them what happened. I was genuinely touched by that moment too as it's rare to find anywhere, but especially at the office. After going back to the office I felt as if I had to escape again or risk that they would gang up on me and carry me back to the hospital. I couldn't tell anyone why I knew I was going to be okay because I didn't know for myself and let's face it; you can't go around telling people that you hear voices in your head. But I had to convince them somehow, and I eventually did.

Later that evening, I called my sister and discussed the "heart attack" with her. My chest was still hurting but it was more of an ache, like after straining a muscle. I was still worried though and the very next day was spent at the cardiologist running a stress test with some kind of dye running through my veins. Let me tell you, that cardiologist was none too happy to be running a stress test on a patient he didn't know, and who had just refused treatment at the hospital. I must have looked like walking trouble, but, he was a Doctor. More importantly, he was a compassionate human being.

He alerted me of the warning signs to watch for during the test and described the entire process at length. He spent a lot of time answering all of my questions to ensure that we were communicating on the same frequency with one another. He took the time and created some space. A habit I have since ingrained in me for when I deal with others in stressful situations.

The testing started very slowly.

I was fine.

He increased the speed.

I was fine.

He raised that incline to where it resembled Kilimanjaro, I looked at him in the eyes, took a couple of deep breaths and blinked when I saw a concerned look on his face. When I inquired as to what so keenly had his interest, he said something like "the incline had the opposite effect as was intended". My heart rate was supposed to increase but instead it decreased a bit. He really didn't want to push me any harder though so he looked at me with a half grin and said "Okay, just hold this for a while and I'll observe you". Apparently I had calmed myself down reflexively to compensate for the added stress.

Eventually, after I sweat enough I guess, he stopped the test. After waiting in the reception area for a while, the nurse started talking to me about when I'd get the results; and that shocked me. This doctor, who had such a great bedside manner, I thought for sure would discuss his thinking before I left. That's when I channeled my mother, as I have often done before when needing to, and started acting like a drill sergeant; believe it or not that is who I get it from.

Five minutes later I found myself interrupting this nice man's lunch as he explained to me that he didn't see anything wrong with me but gave me a stern talking to about smoking cigarettes. I thanked him and left, more puzzled than before, but delighted that I really wasn't going to die; to quote a line from one of my favorite movies, "What the hell?"

Over the next few months, and many doctor visits, I found myself popping pills every morning. I was taking one pill to reduce my blood pressure, another pill to reduce my bad cholesterol, a third pill was an anti-depressant I dubbed my "Happy Pill", a baby aspirin for good measure and allergy medicine. The doctor also insisted I walk around with Nitro, but I blew that one off.

Why an anti-depressant? During a conversation with my sister about our family medical history, we started discussing my mother's condition before she died and it became clear that if my mother were alive today, her condition would be classified as SAD; Social Anxiety Disorder. I recognized some of the symptoms in my past as well. My Doctor was very compassionate when we spoke about these symptoms, and he suggested another pill to lessen those symptoms. An excerpt from Wikipedia on SAD:

Social anxiety disorder (SAD or SAnD), also known as social phobia, is an anxiety disorder which is one of the most common psychiatric disorders. It is characterized by intense fear in social situations, causing considerable distress and impaired ability to function in at least some parts of daily life. While the fear of social interaction may be recognized by the person as excessive or unreasonable, overcoming it can be quite difficult. Social anxiety disorder is known to appear at an early age in most cases. 50% of those who develop this disorder have developed it by the age of 11 and 80% have developed it by age 20. Physical symptoms often accompanying social anxiety disorder include excessive blushing, sweating (hyperhidrosis), trembling, palpitations and nausea. Stammering may be present, along with rapid speech. Panic attacks can also occur under intense fear and discomfort.

I was trying to be very present while discussing SAD with my doctor. I was trying to observe my thoughts, trying to feel my emotions to know what was right for me. Responding to the moment is always better than reacting to the moment as reaction is based on conditioning or preconceived notions, and *their* resulting actions. Responding comes from the moment itself and is usually only what the moment calls for. Practicing this is not always easy however, especially whenever someone labels me, as I have a tendency to react and get defensive-I'm working on that. For instance, when I am assumed to be suffering from SAD, whoever is making that assumption has preconceived notions about that label, and those notions are automatically associated with whatever that label is applied to; in this case me! In a word, it's stereotyping; which is a limiting structure. My ire gets up when anything limiting crosses my path. Labels are limiting. Oh, he has such and such so he can't do that. There are infinite possibilities for what human beings can achieve; regardless of other's preconceived notions.

I used to pick on people close to me for popping pills every day like candy only now I was doing it too, and let me tell you something; it didn't help. Well, at first it was a godsend, but over time, the feeling of residual side effects built up and the symptoms that the drugs were treating, started to return. This happened over time and of course I consulted my Doctor and we tried different medications until one day I found myself arguing with him over who was right, me or him; and this was over a medical issue! My Doctor was fantastic, renown is his field, but just like the priest, he had no answers as to WHY my brain functions this way or my metabolism, or whatever. I'm trying not to be specific about any given supposed ailment but I like to know the root cause of *any* issue and then address it there, not just treat the symptoms. One way I find helpful in getting to the root cause of an issue is to simply ask why? Just like a child would with all the nonjudgmental innocence you can muster. Accept the answer as truth, and then test it again by asking; why? Eventually you will come to one of two ends; belief or disbelief, and you will have worked through all of the options that have come to mind. If you come to disbelief, look elsewhere.

I looked elsewhere.

I got fed up, put on my drill sergeant hat and went on the attack (metaphorically); devoting every free moment I had at my disposal, along with every dollar I had at my disposal, to fixing me so I wouldn't suffer the fate my mother had, and I thought I was destined for. I was going to do whatever it took to get healthy and get off all of these drugs. That was my stated intent. I would research methods that attempt to address the root cause of these issues. I read a lot of books, watched a lot of videos; Google was my friend. Joan Bello has authored many great books but when I found The Benefits of Marijuana: Physical, Psychological and Spiritual by Joan Bello, it was like she had written the book just for me. As I progressed in my research and trials to get healthy, I found that the root cause of my issues was "myself"! "I found my spirituality" is perhaps a better way to put it? I know that sounds new age but I think of a universal power or space *that is* the universe, and that universal space creates everything within, including us. I learned how to sum up very complex topics into bite sized chunks, devoid of any real meaning; for presentations to executives. I think this sentence sums it up nicely. I think of a universal power or space that is the universe, and that space or power creates everything within; including us. So, I don't know what to call it and frankly I hesitate to call it anything, because as soon as I do it's a label. This is where I had to let go, and I mean *really* let go, of what I was always taught to think. This is where you start to break down all barriers to innocent, independent thought and ask "why" until you believe in whatever it is you come to believe. And once you believe it, you'll no longer feel the need to ask why, and you will no longer be troubled by the question.

Faith is the knowledge of your beliefs. Once you sense it and realize how vast it is, you will actually laugh at yourself for thinking you could ever fully grasp it. In that moment, faith, the knowledge of your beliefs, then overwhelms your emotions with blissful joy. That is the feedback from your body you are sensing; your body is trying to tell you that you are on the right track. The knowledge of my beliefs includes the knowledge that there's more than we can comprehend at this stage in our human development. Faith is something you feel emanating from within your own body. It's caused by the understanding of your knowledge, not being able to explain it. Believing in something doesn't mean that you have to be able to explain it; you believe it more than know it with all of your being. You sense its accuracy. It lets you know of its presence by overwhelming your emotions with joy.

After you go through this self-examination and come to a belief, you won't get upset when others scoff or question you, because you'll no longer feel the need to question what you believe; until somebody asks you a question about your beliefs that you haven't yet contemplated. Take no offense still; instead, be grateful and thank the person. Ask yourself the same question before meditation and go down that rabbit hole until you either believe or disbelieve. And then get back to the person who, under normal circumstances would have offended you. Get back with them and explain your reasoning and offer to discuss it over a friendly whatever you do; beer, coffee or, cannabis. Enjoy the discovery with another human being rather than the persona and remain present with them. Admittedly, your mileage may vary, but I prefer to at least try and fail than to not even try at all.

I used this same "asking why" approach while trying to decide about writing this book. It went something like this.

Why write a book about this?

I think my mother sought help in her own way. I did too, in my own way, but if I didn't look at non-traditional or alternative methods, I wouldn't have found anything other than pharmaceuticals and years of therapy. My approach to this awakening has been to maintain presence from a peaceful innocence or more bluntly, peaceful ignorance. I had put off spirituality and inner feelings to work on what I though was more important in my life and genuinely felt as if these religious or spirituality topics were impediments to that endeavor. What did I value more than myself? Well, everything really. My Career, my social status, a nice house, a nice car, death money (401k) etc. I was fat and dumb, but not happy. I changed myself however and wanted to share what worked for me. That's why I wanted to write this book.

Why? I want to share what worked for me because although I went to extremes at times, losing weight and taking back control of your body and mind is easy to accomplish, just not necessarily so with traditional methods; I now realize this only after learning it the hard way as usual. I thought if I write a book about my experience, somebody who is searching for answers may find what I have done useful. That's what it felt like to me many times as I was searching for a specific answer to a question stuck in my head, only to suddenly and mysteriously come upon the answer in a book. I can help with that I thought. Not because this is some new idea, but because I had the audacity to ask myself why again!

Why? Feeling my emotion when asking why this time, my heart made me realize that the right thing to do is tell the whole truth. Complete honesty was necessary to reduce the stigma attached with alternative treatments and medicines; and yes I include cannabis in that category. That's what MY inner being said. But I also realized that to take the stigma off of that, I first had to get through my own male ego and its tendency to bury emotion; in an attempt to break that barrier long enough for men, including this one, to open their hearts a little so as to incorporate new perspectives.

We need to change how we view marijuana / Cannabis, and not just legalize it for recreational use and tax revenue. This plant has many benefits that have been proven for centuries by many different cultures. I'm happy to consider it alternative medicine if it makes the stigma more palatable, but I don't want the benefactors of marijuana to be viewed or treated by society as an outcast for ingesting a plant or weed to be honest. The only way I can try to shape that outcome I thought, was to tell the truth publicly, and under my real name.

You see, I learned what I know about this topic from reading books written by authors who write because they feel compelled to help society in some way; I ended up walking myself through a spiritual awakening with that help. This awakening, <u>I believe</u>, is what has started the repair of my physical body. It started with weight loss, which adjusted everything else. What I wanted to share was how I actually applied these principles I have learned as I believe that most great ideas are never fully realized due to poor implementation; and I can't be truthful without giving credit to Cannabis. I also can't get through to the like-minded thick headed men without breaking through the machismo of the male ego first, and so at times I may sound like a drill sergeant.

I encourage you to seek for yourself, as we are all the same, yet our journeys and experiences in life have been so very different. Do what feels right for your inner being regardless of what your mind, or the mind of others, say. Be non-judgmental of yourself.

THE TIPPING POINT

Before Marijuana Therapy, it seemed like despite whatever I would try to focus on, my mind would prevent me by distracting me with thoughts from the past, or thoughts perceived to be poised to happen in the future. These thoughts would consume me; I would identify with them, and my body would end up in a state of either anxiety or anger. I had assumed I could get another drug like a tranquilizer or something from my doctor, but I wanted off the stuff I was already on at the moment. My health was so bad I thought, I didn't even dare drink a beer because the top of my head would feel like a percolating coffee pot with my skyrocketing blood pressure whenever I drank. Doctors confirmed my fears of bad health which only served to reinforce my anxiety about it. Regardless of how I've tried to refute it, there's simply no way to deny the benefit that meditation and cannabis have had on my ability to lose weight, reduce my blood pressure and fix my cholesterol. Even if for no other apparent reason, or to make it more palatable to believe, Marijuana therapy Calmed me down, allowed me to focus and relaxed me. By allowing me to relax into meditation, I found some inner peace. Finding my inner peace, even a fleeting moment of it, made me want more! More knowledge, more peace. Call it desire, drive or power if you will but I believed that I had the energy to turn my situation around; naturally, and using my inner sense.

I really didn't want to write a book about marijuana, but whoa, those pesky principals of mine kick in and I think that in order for me to tell this story truthfully, I would have to include using cannabis with the hope of taking some of the stigma away. If I didn't include any part of marijuana in this book, someone looking for help by reading this book may not realize the full benefit of what I am describing, because a crucial part of the equation was left out. This natural occurring object called Marijuana or Cannabis, that society has outlawed and given a bad reputation, was used by our ancestors for much the same purpose that I use it today; connectedness. Whenever I try to describe marijuana therapy and how it helped me, I usually get asked the same two questions; how does marijuana therapy actually work and what is vaporization, how do you do it? I really wanted to leave the cannabinoid system to Joan Bello, NORML and others in the field of medicine as I don't want to pass myself off as an expert when I'm not. I will however try to point you in the right direction so you can research and create a list of questions or disbeliefs. You can either come to the conclusion yourself, or discuss this with your doctor when you feel comfortable.

The cannabinoid system is named after the plant that led to its discovery (Cannabis). This internal system is considered to be involved in establishing and maintaining overall human health, communicating through the spinal column. Cannabinoids and their receptors are located in the brain, organs, connective tissues, glands, and immune cells. In each of these, the cannabinoid system performs different tasks, but the goal of the disparate system is the same; balance.

The cannabinoid system attempts to establish and maintain a stable internal environment despite whatever happens in the external environment.

This is an excerpt from NORML:

"Cannabinoids promote this balance throughout the body, from the sub-cellular, to the organism, and perhaps to the community and beyond. Here's one example: autophagy, a process in which a cell sequesters part of its contents to be self-digested and recycled, is mediated by the cannabinoid system. While this process keeps normal cells alive, allowing them to maintain a balance between the synthesis, degradation, and subsequent recycling of cellular products, it has a deadly effect on malignant tumor cells, causing them to consume themselves in a programmed cellular suicide. The death of cancer cells, of course, promotes homeostasis and survival at the level of the entire organism."

Cannabinoids are primarily found between the major organs of the body. Let's say you fall and scrape your knee. This means that around the scrape on your knee, cannabinoids will attempt to decrease the release of activators and sensitizers from the injured tissue, stabilizing the nerve cell to prevent excessive firing, and calm nearby immune cells to prevent release of pro-inflammatory substances. In short, Cannabinoids act as a cushion to minimize the impact of your injury. It attempts to "balance" the injury rather than have you cry out in pain or not feel it at all.

The general thinking is that the Cannabinoid system interacts with our immune system, nervous system, and all of the body's organs, to establish a bridge or the way I think of it, a switch, that then regulates all that passes through it. The spinal column is the back plane of the switch that processes this information. By studying this system, researchers have begun to see glimpses of a physical reason that explains how your state of consciousness can promote health or disease. In other words, negativity in thought and action has a detrimental effect on your health!

Cannabinoid research, primarily happening outside of the US, continues to show links or pointers, to how Cannabinoid system assists with psychotherapy. For instance, some research indicates that the administration of cannabinoids often promotes sharing, humor, and creativity and that cannabinoids may directly influence a person's open-mindedness and ability to move beyond limiting patterns of thought and behavior from past situations. Breaking down barriers to free innocent thought or structures, is critical for removing judgment, negativity and overall genuine happy living; which is a key concept in this book. I energized my cannabinoid system with Cannabis and afterwards I found it much easier to focus and break down the structures that were preventing me from enjoying the moment as it is.

All vertebrate species, those with a spine, have an integrated cannabinoid system that is an essential part of life and adaptation to environmental changes happening around the species. Using genetic comparison of the cannabinoid receptors in these different species, scientists estimate that the cannabinoid system could have evolved in animals over 600 million years ago. Cannabinoid receptors present throughout the human body, embedded in cell membranes, and are believed to be more numerous than any other receptor system! Researchers have only identified two cannabinoid receptors: however CB1, predominantly present in the nervous system, connective tissues, gonads, glands, and organs; and CB2, predominantly found in the immune system and its associated structures. Many tissues contain both CB1 and CB2 receptors, each linked to a different action. Researchers speculate there may be a third cannabinoid receptor waiting to be discovered.

Phytocannabinoids are plant substances that stimulate cannabinoid receptors. Delta-9-tetrahydrocannabinol, or THC, is the most psychoactive and certainly the most famous of these substances, but other cannabinoids such as cannabidiol (CBD) and cannabinol (CBN) are gaining the interest of researchers due to a variety of healing properties. Most phytocannabinoids have been isolated from cannabis sativa, but other medical herbs, such as echinacea purpura, have been found to contain non-psychoactive cannabinoids as well. Cannabinoids have antioxidant properties that protect the leaves and flowering structures of the marijuana plant itself from ultraviolet radiation. These natural cannabinoids neutralize the harmful free radicals generated by UV rays, protecting the cells of the plant. In humans, free radicals cause aging, cancer, and impaired healing. Antioxidants found in plants have long been promoted as natural supplements to prevent free radical harm. Research has shown that small doses of cannabinoids from marijuana can signal the body to make more endocannabinoids and build more cannabinoid receptors. This is why many first-time marijuana users don't "feel" an effect, but by their second or third time using the herb they have built more cannabinoid receptors and their body is ready to respond. More receptors increase a person's sensitivity to cannabinoids which means that after your Cannabinoid system is "charged", smaller doses of medicine will have larger effects, and the individual has an enhanced baseline of endocannabinoid activity. I have experienced this first hand. As cannabis built up in my system, I realized that I needed a lot less on a daily basis to maintain that level of medication, quite contradictory to most manmade pharmaceuticals. I have no doubt that a functional cannabinoid system is essential for good health; I believe it.

My mother didn't smoke, anything; and even though she was a large woman, after drinking half of a beer, she wouldn't even want to drive. She simply didn't use any kind of substance for personal gratification, other than food. If this book were available to her years ago, she *still wouldn't have tried cannabis* because the general consensus was that it's a drug. That stigma needs to end or at least be lessened to a great degree so more people can feel comfortable about using this plant in their daily diet. Times are changing, states are legalizing the use for recreation but I think we need to focus more on the benefits of this plant as a whole and go from there. I also don't trust the Congress or the pharmaceutical lobby to determine how this plant is best used; although I applaud the current administration for not overacting as the country comes to terms with this debate. Elected officials want to be re-elected, pharmaceutical companies focus on shareholder value. Citizens, we the people, must insist on keeping Cannabis natural. Keeping cannabis naturally beneficial and fun for adults, much like a good homebrew; that's my preference. Let's not create a new cigarette-like corporate conglomerate or ultra-condensed pill versions of the plant with so much regulation processing and taxation as to make us stumble forward. Instead, let it progress naturally and openly with minimal interference from profiteers and middlemen. Sure, tax the sale somehow and use that money for something else that the populace needs; but don't get carried away. This plant isn't another type of beer; it's so much more.

Marijuana is a weed, hence the nickname "weed", and as such, is currently native to all continents on the planet but Antarctica. Marijuana is the third most popular recreational drug in America (behind only alcohol and tobacco). Research indicates that Cannabis may be a useful supplement to treatment for: Nerve damage pain relief, nausea, spasticity, glaucoma, and some movement disorders; marijuana's medicinal properties may also protect the body against some types of malignant tumors. NORML is an organization that has been around for a while. The mission statement on their website reads:

*"NORML's mission is to move public opinion
sufficiently to achieve the repeal of marijuana
prohibition so that the responsible use of cannabis
by adults is no longer subject to penalty."*

I completely agree with and support their cause. I used cannabis to help me relax enough to keep the thoughts out of my mind when I meditate, not to go party with. I don't think cannabis is any different than any other tool I might use in this endeavor such as relaxing music, aroma therapy, a steam bath or sex. (Where's Dr. Ruth when you need her?). Sure, there's a high but I'm not a kid anymore who's experimenting. After a while, the high becomes a problem honestly. You are after balance, harmony and peace; not highs and lows. Balance. What you are after is building your internal cannabinoid system back to health and then maintaining that; and that doesn't mean that you're always high either. I think of Cannabis as nature's allergy pill for the heart, soul and inner being.

You, the sufferer, first have to be open enough to trust yourself. Don't trust me, trust yourself. Sometimes a realization or "awakening" can happen with a suggestion or pointer from something external, but for those of us thick headed types, life is more than capable of throwing us a wallop of a nightmare to deal with and learn from. So do yourself a favor, and start looking at your "problems" as lessons, so as to *lessen*, the amount of wallops life throws your way. Look at an apparent problem or issue as a life lesson to be used as growth. Learn from it what you can; ask why? If you find that it's too painful to think about, or you simply can't focus, talk to your doctor about the use of focus enhancing supplements and or cannabis. Personally, I wanted to keep it natural so I didn't explore the various pharmaceutical methods. I certainly wasn't very patient either so therapeutic treatment over a period of time didn't seem like a feasible option. I probably also didn't have the option for medicinal use of cannabis as a kind of psychotherapy enhancement. It's not on the approved list of ailments that medicinal marijuana is permitted to be used for in many if not all the states anyway. This by the way is despite a whole lot of research and successful trials of using marijuana in the 1960's to assist in psychotherapy treatment.

Thankfully, I have forgotten the probably minor events of that day which was the tipping point that got my head percolating again, but the events made me determined to fix my Self. Those very same nerve-wracking symptoms had resurfaced through all of the pharmaceutical drugs I was taking. I felt horrible physically, and tormented mentally. In my mind, I needed a beer, or six, but drinking when your body struggles under normal activity, is not a good idea. This is also why the normal exercise programs people swear by didn't appeal to me; I had to lose weight before I started exercising, and I needed to stop eating my emotions in order to lose weight. If I could just relax…

I knew a guy who knew a guy; you know?

Actually, with all the buzz about medicinal marijuana, it must have just been in my head but I started wondering if it would be worth the trouble of trying to get a prescription. But, really? I can't just walk into my doctor's office and say hey, how about some pot? Just say no right? Anyone remember the TV commercial, this is your brain (I think it was an uncracked egg), then the hand would crack it into a frying pan and the announcer would say, this is your brain on drugs. At 41, I felt I needed the few brain cells I had left. I had a great youth you see, and I certainly didn't feel the need for any more "experimentation". This is the stigma associated with using cannabis today. Then I started doing some research and I came across that very thick but well referenced book: The Benefits of Marijuana: Physical, Physiological and Spiritual, by Joan Bello. I urge you to get that book and read through it at least once; then use it too, as a reference.

I knew a guy who knew a guy; remember?

I decided to "test" my theory by getting high on marijuana for the first time in a long while. Honestly, I felt as if I had nothing to lose; this was my body and I was going to do whatever I needed to do to make it healthy again. Of course, I had caveats to that objective. I needed to do whatever I needed to do, but without any activity I consider exercise; no dieting, no drugs, nothing unpleasant. Nobody thought I could do it but they wouldn't say so. Instead, all you hear is how you need to diet and exercise. I remember a time in the service where the weather was too cold to perform our morning physical training outside as per usual. As we started smiling at the news, our sergeant started smiling back and telling us we were going to do some yoga jazzercise stuff with the women instead; inside the gym. Let me tell you, the women were laughing in the end as we all flopped about on the floor no longer able to move. That impressed me then and so I looked it up again and fell in love with yoga. There are all kinds of yoga and I would take from what felt right in each of them and incorporate it into my routine; staring by just trying to balance on one foot. That was the beginning of action meditation for me and permitted my first purposeful glimpse into union; which provided me the confidence to move forward but only after I was medicated.

Prior to cannabis, I was had been trying to meditate by sitting still; but failing. Stillness with no thought was my goal. The longest time I managed to perform my version of meditative yoga, I call it Yogatate, was for 6 minutes, before being overwhelmed by frustration. That's six minutes of meditative yoga, having a thought and letting it go, back to the meditation of awareness on your pose or posture and breathing; on and on, shifting back and forth until frustration. Six minutes was my longest time to be able to "Yogatate" as I called it, before cannabis. After Cannabis was built up in my system however, I was meditating and doing yoga peacefully for an hour or so every weekend day and sometimes during the week. This just felt right to me despite any advice to the contrary and once I had realized some of the benefits, I doubled my efforts.

Let's be honest; at first, I got high and played video games. That was fun for a week, but then when the same frustrating situations, emotions and issues would seemingly repeat themselves, I was still dealing with them the same way. This can't be, I thought. I must be doing something wrong. Why aren't I relaxed and groovy? Asking that question of myself did the trick. Asking myself why, before an at home, make-shift weekend long meditation retreat, while medicated with cannabis. And after lots of walking, yoga, and meditation over the course of that weekend, I was able to dig deep and get to the root cause.

What that weekend taught me most, was a process; how to take a thought, and work it through in such a way as to let my brain give "processor time" to a thought or question, and then drop the question without further allocated time, but after feeling the emotion; if any. If there were an emotion, I would then focus on where I felt that emotion and why. This is when I started to study the energy system or "the Chakras "of human beings. There are seven major chakras associated with the human body. These major chakras do not actually exist as "objects" (they are actually energy patterns) but there are certain specific locations on the body that correspond to them, five along the spine, and two on the head. Each chakra is shaped like a funnel or whirlpool of energy. Their vortices lie inside the body, along the spinal cord (which corresponds to our central energy switch) and up into the head.

The chakras are described as being aligned in an ascending column from the base of the spine to the top of the head. In various traditions chakras are associated with multiple physiological functions, an aspect of consciousness, a classical element, and other distinguishing characteristics.

23

The chakras are thought to vitalize the physical body and to be associated with interactions of a physical, emotional and mental nature. They are considered the location of life energy or prana, also called shakti, qi (Chinese; ki in Japanese), koach-ha-guf[21] (Hebrew), bios (Greek) & aether (Greek, English), which is thought to flow among them, along pathways called nadis. The function of the chakras is to spin and draw in this energy to keep the spiritual, mental, emotional and physical health of the body in balance. They are said by some to reflect how the unified consciousness of humanity (the immortal human being or the soul), is divided to manage different aspects of earthly life (body/instinct/vital energy/deeper emotions/communication/having an overview of life/contact to God). The chakras are placed at differing levels of spiritual subtlety, with Sahasrara at the top being concerned with pure consciousness, and Muladhara at the bottom being concerned with matter, which is seen simply as condensed, or gross consciousness.

For a practical example, anxiety is usually felt in my chest or heart-mind (Anahata), fear in my stomach area (Swadhisthana). When unrest is felt in a chakra that usually indicates a blockage of energy. This was how I determined if a structure or preconceived notion was preventing me from enjoying the moment. If there were a blockage of energy associated with a thought, then that structure needs to go. There are two sides to everything, yin and yang, positive and negative, love and trust on one side, fear and doubt or anxiety on the other. If I were to focus on loving and trusting more, maybe my fear and doubt will go away I thought; it does. But facing your fears and anxieties only means accepting them, I had learned, and that means to accept yourself as you are; this moment.

Here's a practical example of acceptance. I just stepped outside to enjoy a not so socially acceptable drug; a cigarette. As other people were walking around, I found myself getting that anxious feeling in my chest again; as soon as I noticed it I asked why? Why was I anxious? Then I realized it was because I have perceived that people think smoking is bad and only bad people smoke. I had identified myself with that conditioned thinking and my emotions kicked in. With that realization I smiled a bit, relaxed into the moment and finished my smoke knowing that I am not that cigarette.

With cannabis in my system, I feel as if I can finally focus long enough to feel my body, but also mentally clear enough to not get wrapped up in my thoughts. The more cannabis I consumed over time, the more it built up in my system and the better it became; just like an allergy pill. Furthermore, the more it built up in my system, the more relaxed and groovy I remained throughout the day. I was liking these results so I did it more and more, until it became a nightly meditative practice I dubbed Cannabis and Coffee.

First let me say that I don't smoke or eat marijuana. I have done both in the past and there are some very good recipes that eliminate the high but leave the medicine. By far however, the new and improved manner to consume cannabis is by vaporization. The concept is to blow dry hot air across the plant and into a bag that you then inhale and release. Different cannabinoids activate at different temperatures so if you can get an accurate vaporizer, and they are commercially available, you can sort of "tune" the usage a bit and eliminate or minimize the carcinogens that come from burning it. Herbal marijuana is thought to contain over one hundred different cannabinoids, including THC, which all work synergistically to produce better medical effects and less side effects than the THC synthesized counterparts available today. Scientific inquiry and patient testimonials both indicate that herbal marijuana has superior medical qualities to synthetic cannabinoids. Medical marijuana could become a component of preventative medicine, and a dietary supplement for our increasingly toxic, carcinogenic environment. This is not a new concept as it was well known to the indigenous medical practice of ancient India and China and probably more.

The VOLCANO Vaporization System http://www.storz-bickel.com/vaporizer/vaporizing-application-herbs.html

Over time as cannabis built up in my system, my love of yoga and meditation grew to where I completely stopped playing video games and watching any TV. My ritual was to come home from the office, greet the pets, make a pot of coffee and sit down at the computer, ingest cannabis while researching whatever I was into at the moment and drink coffee (Beatnik anyone?). Then, I would Yogatate, take the dog for a meditation walk of at least one mile (later these became quite elaborate meditative walks), return, shower and have a yogurt with granola; my substitution for a nightly bowl of ice cream. At that time, I was having only coffee for breakfast and juicing for lunch with coffee or tea for dinner and a light meal or healthy snack before bed. You could call that a diet but I wouldn't want you to. This is what worked for me at the time I was trying to cleanse. I have since learned more about the proper fuels required for the human body to accomplish certain tasks like losing fat while toning muscle. This wasn't a rigid practice either; I experimented. If I wanted pizza one day, I would have pizza. Got a craving for chips? No problem; eat a whole bag. And I would, and I would feel miserable. That's success. When you eat something and you hear your body say yummy or yuck, you can then modify what you give it. You of course have to be able to hear your body, which also means to understand or comprehend your body first; and that didn't come to me until after I started practicing body awareness meditation.

Using this analytical process, I was able to get through enough conditioning to start making real progress toward better overall health. It's also how I gauged what and how much to fuel my body; and you know what? Today, if I don't get my chard juice, I have a tendency to get cranky.

About meditation; there are many good books that can describe how to meditate and the various forms of meditation much better than I. Davidji's book, Secrets of Meditation, is probably my personal favorite, but I have researched and experimented with many types just like I did with yoga. I then mix and match until I feel I have a routine that is right for me. How do you know if it's right for you? If you feel that it's beneficial to you, if it brings you peace somehow and you think you can do it forever than that's your practice; lean into it. My personal version of meditation is no longer stationary or sedate. I meditate while doing yoga, walking, and shopping. I try to view life as one big meditation with the focus being love, trust and peaceful existence stemming from the present moment. I warned you about my hippy tendencies.

If this would be your absolute "first time you have ever tried meditation" moment, and you were really hoping I would provide some advice, try this; sit in a comfortable place and in a comfortable position. Ready? Sit!

Now, hold that; just sit still. If a thought comes into your head, try to recognize it as a thought coming into your head **instead of *reacting*** to the thought that came into your head. That's how it begins. From there, you get better and better at recognizing your thoughts, and then your emotions and then you realize that you are the observer of yourself. With continued practice you will be able to determine if you want to allow the thought some "processor time", as I call it, in your mind. You can then decide to discard the thoughts as they enter if you wish and just be at peace. If the focus of your meditation is to simply be, to sit still with yourself, than all you need to do, when you recognize a thought, is to discard it and let it go, shift your awareness back to the present moment. Now you are meditating.

What? Yes, it's that simple. So what's the focus of you meditation? No thoughts. Just be; just sit, stand, walk, talk or whatever it is. Just be in the moment. Present awareness.

A goal of mine during this period was to meditate twice per day; once in the morning and once in the evening. I chose dawn and dusk because I feel more energized at those times, more connected somehow. My morning meditation never included cannabis unless I was going to watch a sunrise with the dog while meditating or something similar on the weekend. All other times during meditation I have found that cannabis is a crucial component to relaxing the mind enough to stay with the moment and focus. I know I'm not the first to mention how much focus cannabis provides but, I've lost around 100 pounds in around one year which helped to correct my blood pressure and cholesterol and I eventually stopped taking my happy pill and allergy medication. Four pills gone by one plant. Let me say that again, I successfully stopped taking all medication except for cannabis and I'm feeling great! I call that a focus enhancing plant.

The weight loss enabled me to become more active in a way I find to be enjoying; meditative walking. It also allowed me to explore more advanced Power Yoga. Both healthy activities have started to tone my body back into shape and has definitely restored my flexibility, which has resulted in even more weight loss. All of this was made possible, because my meditation practice showed me a peaceful existence inside me, which grew with each meditation and increased my desire to learn more, which helped me to ask why, to the point of breaking down barriers. Breaking down barriers or structures has made me look at the world anew, such as a child, and has reduced my supposed symptoms of SAD. Meditation has opened my mind and cleansed my spirit, but cannabis is what allowed me to be able to meditate. All drugs, except for cannabis, which is a plant and not a drug regardless of what labels people want to associate with it, have been out of the picture for a while now with me; and every day only gets better. I don't even have allergy issues anymore. Meditation, a plant based diet, healthy non-jarring exercise and cannabis is how I primarily balance myself now; although during this exploration, I tried many other activities as well, like fasting. My second weekend long fasting retreat is when I went deep with meditation for the first time. Deep not only as in the mind but also the body and spirit. It was union and it was bliss. It's when I first felt peace.

I started this journey with Yoga by standing on one foot.

When I would try sitting still and I recognized a thought had taken my attention away from the focus of my meditation,

I would let my body move freely into yoga like moves and work out the thought or emotion. Kim Eng teaches this kind of meditation. The idea is to let your body work out your emotions and thoughts that flow through you as they happen. To feel and release; like catch and release if you've been fishing before. I had one small problem however; I would sit down, get comfortable, and immediately start break dancing. No kidding, I shared it with someone long after it happened, when I was comfortable enough to discuss it, and he agreed; it looked like break dancing. That's what my mind and emotions were like at that time but how was I to know that? All I had seen was an online video of Kim doing these lovely Tai Chi like moves; I looked like a reject from the eighties.

"No Judging" as Kim is fond of saying.

The focus of your meditation is ultimately nothing, but to make it easier to wrap our heads around, let's start by simply paying all of your attention to breathing. You really don't have to do anything other than sit still and pay attention to your breathing. That's all they say there is to meditating, the proverbial "they" is correct but…. what if that's not peaceful? My answer is to add cannabis.

I added music and it got somewhat better but there really isn't a secret. Persistence pays off with meditation; you just have to keep at it. Cannabis allowed my mind to focus which can be of great help in both yoga and meditation. Focusing on the object of your meditation or the yoga pose while breathing with all your being, not just a slice of it, is what union is all about to me. After continuing to practice for weeks, I started to slowly notice my breaths were slower and fuller, my pace had slowed, and there was more concentration and less chatter in my head. I began to feel again. A smile, or in military parlance, a shit eating grin, was almost a permanent fixture on my face. I kept at it. Every morning, every evening. All weekend. Reading, meditating and yoga; all with cannabis. Then, that one Sunday evening when I went deep, into a peaceful, quiet loving sensation of union, I worked through some emotional blockage or baggage…..

…. and then burst out crying like a baby.

Since then, I haven't relented. I have been using my surroundings to work through my thoughts and emotions with a healthy dose of twice daily meditation, daily meditation walking, and a much more natural, plant based diet which includes juicing and cannabis. The Cannabis in my diet is to maintain the levels of the relevant cannabinoids in my blood so I don't need to "get high" to meditate. I don't want to be high; I want to be relaxed and groovy. There is a difference that you can feel after it has built up in your system and all you need to do is maintain that level.

What did I find as the root cause that made me cry like a baby? The honest answer is that I found myself, but that answer will be interpreted, confusingly. What happened is that I saw myself for what I am; probably for the first time in a long while. I saw all of my flaws and accepted them. I evaluated what I thought were my strengths only to realize that I had a completely different and seldom used capability that was much greater than any of my perceived strengths; and that was my capability to love. Okay, male ego breaking time. There is more to the word love than you think. When you see something in the world that you are positive is, or is supposed to be a certain way, with parameters that are absolute; you

31

have just judged with a preconceived notion, or stereotyped the situation. Yes you have. There are no absolutes! There is only the present moment and what it contains.

What if there were a person involved or affected and you just passed judgment on them? We are all human, we are all here together. We are all the same, but often times with different issues, roles or appearances. That person you just passed judgment on is another human soul, another essence, another energy field. You have no idea what kind of day they've had in their worldly existence today. Where's your humility? Where's your compassion? Where's your connectedness? Where's your *love*?

Anytime you judge something, anything, with a preconceived notion or anytime you react, or oftentimes overreact, in a pre-determined manner rather than responding in the moment; you are neither humble, compassionate nor loving. Love each other with no preconceived notions as your default position in life. Try that kind of unconditional love toward everyone my friend and I trust your ego will enjoy the challenge; if it's up to it.

There are many "normal" ways to address procrastination or to dig deep into your soul to see what's going on. But normal and patience are not common descriptors of my actions. Years of therapy while I live a miserable partial existence isn't my idea of help I'm sorry to say. I say partial because the pharmaceuticals definitely had an impact on me; dulling my senses. I liken this type of treatment to getting allergy shots.

I have been told I have allergies; another limiting structure. Turns out, you only have allergies if you believe you have allergies. Otherwise, you may just have a stuffy nose for the moment that deserves a good breath or two to clear out those cobwebs. My allergy test results reported that of all things, I was allergic to dust and animal hair the most. I live with a dog and a cat and where isn't there dust? Modern Medicine's cure is to, slowly over time, inject me with what I'm allergic to so my body will build up a tolerance to it. This process is measured in years by the way. I reminded the good doctor that I already live with my allergies, Java the mini Aussie and Tofu the kitty and I didn't think I needed more allergens in my blood to make me feel miserable for the next few years, while I try and medicate against what you're artificially injecting into me.

It's hard to describe sometimes but, when restless and ranting, my mind was like a game of "pile on" that maybe you played when you were a kid. Your thoughts just keep going and going, unconsciously. This adds layer upon layer of thoughts, which create worries, which manifests itself as fear, which paralyzes you into procrastination. That's my version of Humania; a term coined by Steve Taylor to describe the "normal" neurosis that affects almost everyone.

It's that simple.

Great but now what?

This is where meditation comes in.

Seriously, I'm not advocating anything more than sitting still. Maybe a little chanting or breathing if the moment calls for it; relax and get into it. What I'm saying is that the absolute first thing you must do is clear your mind and relax by any means possible. Clear your mind and your ass will follow. I said that for years because I thought it was catchy but I never really listened to it; until now. Forget all judgments; whatever works for you is good enough, but be mindful and use your inner being to guide you. Once you find your way, whatever healthy combination of techniques works for you, you'll be able to sit still and enjoy the moment or take a walk and be present with the moment as it is; peacefully. If you do find an activity or non-activity that provides you this peace, repeat it, over and over again until there's no effort to it anymore. That's your meditation practice. Then it becomes the basis for everything else you do. In order for me to be able to meditate I needed to first learn to free my mind of thoughts. Music was a help at first, then a hindrance. Reading in silence was blissful, for a while, but then inevitably the thoughts would fill my consciousness again. I found that after I started medicating with Cannabis, the cannabinoid system in my body responded, and Yogatat'ing was the easiest method for clearing my mind of negative thoughts, or thought about the future or past. Picture me slapping myself on the forehead; it turns out that all you need to do to clear your mind, is to create a little space in your life, sit still and stretch.

When thoughts come into my mind, I now find myself questioning them. I question their motive before I let my mind concentrate on them. My goal is to be aware of my thoughts, not to stop them, but also not to let them have any processor time of my consciousness, unconsciously. Be aware and understand them for what they are and feel the emotions they create throughout my body; so I can then use that feedback to alter both my life and my body toward the way I want it to be. Don't react to the thoughts or emotions going through you, simply pay attention to them and understand them from a place of peaceful innocence. Mindfulness is what this is sometimes referred to as I understand it. By being aware before processing the thought and corresponding emotion, you get to decide what to do with it; this is how you can use it for your benefit. Stop the judgmental thoughts from driving who you are and practice looking at the world from an innocent child's perspective.

How Do I Sit Still?

Uh, excuse me, can you please show me how to sit still?

What did you just feel after reading that question? That's what it feels like when you can't simply sit and be. That's your first barrier to break down; why can't you sit still and simply be right there, as you are, in this very moment with no thought; just present awareness.

Relaxing was something altogether different for me. It was easy to blame "the job". Substitute whatever you blame your issues on: spouse, parents, school, teacher, coworkers or boss; you get the idea. Let me tell you plainly, I don't care, it's a copout. Look inside yourself first. Too often we get trapped into thinking that the external world needs to change, or that we need to change something external to us in our life. I'm not saying there isn't a problem in your life, I'm saying your procrastination for addressing it comes from within, just like mine did. Address the reasons why you're procrastinating. Do you know?

In my own case, I simply couldn't feel emotions in my body. I had never allowed myself to really feel emotions to begin with and because of that, I couldn't "sense" which direction was right for me. I had my emotions locked away tight, all bottled up. Everything was buried deep, since childhood, when I was first told that big boys don't cry. Just one example of the many seemingly innocent structures applied to us over the years. You see the limiting labels or structures that we live our lives with don't have to stem from anything "bad", just the "normal" will suffice nicely. Yeah, of course you realize that as an adult big boys do indeed cry, but the condition sticks with you and your unconscious mind uses that condition as a rule to live by. That's a structure; a conditioning. Structures and conditions are what is used when we judge people, places, things or situations. If you saw me blubbering in the street, you might react in a judgmental manner to it due to that conditioning. You may not overtly act, like pointing and laughing or ridiculing me as I blubber away, but the thought that enters your head will be rife with your own preconceived notions of men showing emotion publicly. If you can be present long enough to catch yourself before judging a situation however, you can isolate the structure. That structure is what you need to work on by asking why until you come to belief or disbelief. The process of asking why, is what allows you to work through your emotions and release them. I have released knots in various places of tissue throughout my body this way; by releasing emotions while doing yoga. This is also how you will be able to determine right action. I thought about calling this book "The power of Why", after reading the power of "Now" by Eckhart Tolle, as I think asking why is the next logical step after you are in the now.

Let me put it like this; there are two of you. Your persona or ego and then there is that inner being, the true self, the inner child. I prefer to use the word persona as too many, especially in the corporate world, have preconceived notions of what ego means, and those notions stand in the way of true meaning. The role that you play in life is your persona. However you identify yourself, be it as a father, mother, executive, student, son, daughter, blue collar, and white collar, white, black, Latino, Asian and so many more; however you identify, that is your role in life or your persona. I've heard that over ninety nine percent of humans are consumed by their persona. I don't know how that number could be accurate because I can't logically see how the statistics could be accurately derived. Regardless, my point is that the "normal" way most people go through life is what is causing them their problems.

Do this for one day; have no negative thoughts. If I were to now say "Trust me it's not easy", that would be a negative thought. That thought would have come from my persona, not my inner being. Your persona comes from your mind but your **_self_**, your inner being, comes from your heart; hence the phrase 'listen to your heart'. Remember, your mind has built limitations or structures for you over the course of your life. Any thought that you have like, 'I can't do that' or, 'I'm not good enough' or even 'maybe one day', those are all negative thoughts that emanate from your mind with all of those preconceived notions or structures that limit you. So go ahead and just pay attention to all of the negative thoughts that you can throughout the day tomorrow. Then, the next time you meditate, hopefully tomorrow evening, think about how many and how varied those negative thoughts were. That's what's been holding you back; your own mind. Here's the wonderful catch though, now that you know that, you have the upper hand. Why? Glad you asked that question. You will start to notice life a bit clearer, the absurdity of some moments will start standing out a bit more. This is a good thing that starts to happen to someone at the beginning of awakening to the realization of presence. With presence comes power or energy that can spread to others and come back to you. What you have to do is be aware enough to make sure that you are only putting out what you want back.

If you think you can't, that will radiate outwards and come back as you're right; you can't.

If you think decisively with belief and commitment, I am, as in "I am going to lose 100 pounds and get off these pharmaceuticals", guess what? You will; but you have to believe it. Balls to bones, so to speak. I'm not empowering you, you are empowering your **Self.**

Cannabis, over time, will reduce inflammation throughout your body, and enhance your breath; according to well-known documented research. Prana, is a Sanskrit word generally interpreted as life force and breath. I practiced formal breath exercises after medicating with Cannabis, which I would then match to music, and later combine it with yoga. This was how I felt I could best use cannabis, then I realized that it allowed me to relax and simply be; and meditate. Then I combined it into walking and on and on it went.

I needed to first be able to relax physically, before I could quite literally feel my body from within. I wanted to do this so I could identify the emotion that was associated with whatever thought I was having as this is important in determining whether you should take that thought seriously, because it stems from the peace within (right action), or to blow it off as mind chatter trying to distract you (humania).

After I clarified my theory to myself, I needed to state my intent to put it in motion. I stated my intent to drop my weight and increase my cardiovascular activity and then get off the drugs when I felt it was safe. Pam Grout's book E-Squared is great. She opened my eyes to using our energy to accomplish our goals.

I made a conscious decision to change my:

Dietary efforts: I will eat a more natural and plant based diet. I will control portion sizes and change how I eat to include how I look at food.

Activity: I will stick with my mandatory exercise, and find new three new ways to get active.

Spirit: I will research a path of spirituality and find my beliefs. I will remain present. I will make Conscious efforts to relax by vaporizing cannabis.

When I started I was fat, stressed, and full of negativity. My goal was not weight loss but rather health, peace and positive thinking. In other words, I set out to turn it around. I did not have the intention to become a beach body stud muffin. I was simply after peace and health. Those who I consider close to me and to whom I love dearly, now have less patience with my development than I do. No kidding, I used to get daily, unsolicited, passionate advice for how to muscle up or get cut. People were stopping to ask me how much I've lost so far and if I were going to make a video or if I were taking pictures? Honestly, for the first month or so, I didn't even realize I was losing weight. It wasn't until my clothes wouldn't stay on anymore that I suddenly realized it was working. I guess that's why I feel as if I'm in no rush, this is so effortless! Actually, as my flab diminishes I realized a thought in my head was actually worried that if I lost all of my flab, nobody would know I had lost a lot of weight, and I wouldn't be able to "identify" with being someone who has just lost a lot of weight.

That is how a SAD mind thinks. It's also a part of the Egoic Humania I suspect. I laughed that thought away.

I honestly thought that if I could calm my mind enough to have some peace, I could figure this out. Yoga I knew meant mind body and spirit and so I started with that. Most yoga is like a workout session however; sacrificing the spirit and mind for just the body. I started absorbing whatever I could by reading about yoga instead and then adopting what felt right to me. This led me to reading about meditation and then I stopped to regain focus and put it all together. This is what I recommend to others; forget about being rigid in your meditation and yoga practice. Find what works for you and then stick with it. If you feel yourself getting bored, then step it up a notch maybe with longer time spent holding the poses or more strenuous types of poses but always focus on the pose, the moment, your breath. When your mind wanders, gently bring yourself back to your focus. Rinse and repeat.

Meditation brings me closer to nature somehow, and nature calms me. Social Anxiety Disorder or SAD insinuates a fear of social gatherings. My mother had issues going into shopping malls. She would get irritable and frustrated; anxious. Somewhere in my thirties, I started having the same issues. It started as I walked up to the door of the mall, my heart rate would quicken. I would start sweating. I would feel as if everyone inside the mall was watching me having these feelings, everyone somehow felt connected to me. When I walked into an area full of people, my presence would draw everyone's attention. I rationalized this as something known as Command Presence; "The exhibition of personal magnetism or charisma in a leader, the acquisition or development of which tends to promote an aura of authority." A neat little trick I learned in the service for my ego or persona. Now however, I'm not so sure my little trick of reminding myself of my command presence when anxiety struck did anything but prolong my agony. I have command presence yes, for multiple reasons, but that's from a peaceful state, not an anxious one. What I believe is that we are all connected, and our thoughts do indeed project outward. I have also felt a presence in my life for quite some time, but never could nail it down until recently, and now I think I am simply sensitive to the various energies of others. Before I walk into any public place where I used to get anxious, I scan my body first to make sure I'm present. Just a quick wiggle of the toes to feel them and remind myself of my root to the earth. Then I'll scan up my and through my body just to see what I'm feeling. If I do feel anxious, I simply let that emotion be for a moment, feeling it fully and then going back to the moment. I have yet to encounter a time where the feeling hasn't diminished within a couple of minutes and most of the time, that little exercise puts me into a great mood with that grin on my face again. You really don't feel as if there is anyone to talk to about this however; so you start to feel alone, you start to repress it and get back to "real life"; just like when I was a kid. Only after 41 years of this nonsense, life gives you a swift kick in the ass and starts yelling at you, hoping you'll wake up.

Animals and plants are somehow life; I think we can all agree with that. Humans are also life; I think we can all agree with that too. So I look at the world this way; I slept on the Appalachian Trail alone one very fine evening in my twenties. Just me and nature and it was absolutely fantastic. No fear or concerns at all; but I break into a sweat going into a shopping mall? Okay, so if I'm not afraid of life, what am I afraid of? Anxiety is fear. Why was I afraid? I suspect that my own mind was feeding me these thoughts that created the anxiety and either it really was some kind of fear disorder or it was everyone else's thoughts or feelings that I was sensing. I honestly don't know. I don't need to know either because of my faith in not knowing everything. I understand that there is only so much I can understand right now; and seeing as I no longer have those symptoms when I'm present, I simply stay present whenever I feel anxious. It's not that easy at first and it takes practice, but it only improves over time.

I understand what I feel a little bit now and I've opened my heart quite a bit; I let myself trust enough to have faith in other humans again. I gave myself permission to forgive all grudges, held internally or external. This was another stated intent. These results were not granted with instant gratification, but rather with persistence, meditation and cannabis. Why? Did cannabis have an enhancing affect that finally let me see the light? Did it slow me down enough to see the world as it really is, long enough to come to terms with it? My answer would be yes on both counts.

A pill may be derived from plants but processing, while sometimes beneficial, is also destructive at the same time and mileage varies. A plant is a plant. My goal was to try and stay natural, heal my body and ease my mind. Marijuana, I believe, enhances your ability to be aware by increasing your focus. If you treat life as a meditation and your focus is peace, love and happiness, guess what happens when you add something to enhance your focus? This sounds simple enough for me to believe and keeping that enhancement pure and natural allows it to be used to great effect. Cannabis meets those requirements.

After a recent meditation, I remembered a time when I had a very unusual experience while alone, and high, in the Pine Barrens of New Jersey; which is where I spent my teenage years. I was fond of nature and solitude and would often walk the fire lanes of the barrens alone. I found it to be very peaceful and I believe now that I was kind of meditating while walking; until it scared the living daylights out of me one day. That's when I first heard my inner voice; while alone in the middle of the Pine Barrens. I was sixteen maybe? Can you imagine?

For the life of me I wish I could remember what the voice said. The boogie man is what popped into my head followed by the Jersey Devil. That's what I remember. I ran my backside off, racing to get home not knowing what was chasing me and afterwards, I decided that there was nobody I could tell that story to without being ridiculed. At sixteen, I thought I had many other much more important things to occupy my attention, and so I decided to figure it out another day and filed it for later thought.

This is that, much, later thought.

When I meditated again as an adult, the same experience happened but this time I recognized that I was merely present with my thoughts and emotions. Those sensations I interpret as voices were my own. I could actually feel my body and emotions again and hear my thoughts, if only briefly. When I set off to learn more, I found that there appears to be an awakening of consciousness around the world. More and more people are commonly sharing the same language about events that used to only be discussed with near death victims; or people at the time of their death. I seem to feel that it's more akin to evolution of the human species, and I suspect it will be the hallmark of this century; like the eighteenth century is often cited as the birth of modern industrialization; I don't wish to label this however.

Approach to Better Mind Body and Spirit

I'm not advising you to do *any* of this. I think you must listen to your own body and inner being and do what feels right for you. I simply wanted to include what I did with the hope of that it gives you some ideas and maybe remove some stigma about using Cannabis in your routine.

For some reason when I decided to kick this into high gear, I suddenly felt the need to first cleanse my body; naturally. So, I decided to fast over the weekends eating only enough to keep from falling out and try shrink my stomach a bit in the process; it worked. That was my inner being or inner voice that provided me that guidance I had assumed. This is how I approached addressing this journey; to bring balance to my mind body and spirit. I would relax, breathe, and do some light yoga with maybe some relaxing music. You can add some aromatherapy if you want to go wild but also feel free to include cannabis vaporization. You're not trying to have a trippy experience, pay attention; drink coffee if you must. I started ingesting cannabis just before dinner so the high would rapidly dissipate. This also makes what some may think of as "boring food" much more enjoyable too as Cannabis enhances your senses; including your taste buds. Your goal is to observe your thoughts, emotions and physical body all at the same time. You are the observer. Combined with my version of fasting, I considered this to be mini retreat weekends that I would allow myself to have; that gave my male persona permission to try new things with guilt free experimentation. During these weekends, I started reading about vegan and vegetarian diets and their associated health benefits because I needed to learn about various foods if I were going to make them key in my strategy for going natural with no drugs.

I wasn't going to diet, I wasn't going to work out. I was going to get more active and try to consume only natural plant based foods. It was a change of mind forever, not a temporary state. Not a goal. That's how to really set intent. Change what you think, break down your barriers that prevent you from having an open mind.

Activity—Setting myself up for mandatory activity was genius I thought but it quickly turned out to be insufficient for the energy I soon had available. You see, I loathe exercise. I mean I find it unnatural to spend time indoors sweating on an artificial road next to other sweaty people on similar but different artificial roads who, in the name of politeness, never take their attention away from themselves. I did so many push up's, sit up's and ran so far in the Army, that the only way you'll see me run today is if there is someone behind me with a gun. If you see me doing a push up or sit up it's because I fell and I'm simply getting up off the ground. There are forms of exercise that I thoroughly enjoy too; I "force marched" in formation with many others for miles and miles and loved it in the Army. That's when large size groups of troops walk, very fast, with fully loaded back packs for twenty miles or so. After I got out of the Army I was missing that hiking, so in my twenties I hiked along the southern length of the Appalachian Trail. That's exercise I can get into; but it's not common enough in everyday life. So I moved into an apartment on the third floor and got a puppy, Java, whom I adore; forced activity.

Mind you, while I'm watching what I was eating, training a puppy and working, I really started devoting my time to this effort. No more TV except maybe a bit before bed. I stopped watching the news altogether. I even stopped playing video games. I was totally immersed in finding a way to clear my mind that I once even forgot to eat. If not for the grumbling stomach and weak feeling...... that gave me an idea.

A coworker and I were discussing diet stuff and he made me realize that what I needed to change was how I look at food. In my mind, food was to be enjoyed. It was used for celebration and yes, of course it kept us alive. I needed to stop thinking about food as something to be enjoyed BECAUSE it was *stopping me from eating differently*. I never thought I could enjoy vegetables, so I never really tried. I would look at natural leafy vegetables and turn my nose up. I honestly didn't know the names of more than a few vegetables let alone what to do with them; but yet I knew that's what I should be consuming. Juicing, I suspect, was designed for men like me; who mainly gravitate toward eating meat and potato type meals. It's simple and fun to see what you can come up with in a juice and as long as it's all good produce, you really can't do anything wrong with it.

Juicing—My juice makes one eight ounce glass that I drink right away. This one glass of pure natural goodness provides me more vitamins and nutrients than the "normal" food I was eating three times a day. I take half or a whole stalk of chard, three or four kale stems, one big collard green leaf, one stalk of celery, one third of a cucumber and one carrot. To sweeten; one orange or half a lemon and always a green apple, or two if you like it thinner.

I had no idea what Chard, Kale or Collard Greens looked like but when I researched the health benefits, it sounded like something I should be eating. I tried salads, stir fry etc. You *can* make this taste good when cooking; but enough butter can make anything taste good. Taste however, is not why we're eating. <u>Sustenance and brain fuel is why we eat. Not celebration, not enjoyment, not to feel better.</u> I tried to tell myself this as I choked down the first few juices I concocted but after a while, I found this combination that I actually now look forward to and very much enjoy drinking. I suggest you experiment with different ingredients instead of using a recipe book only because I think you will learn more that way.

Routine—Twenty one days, some say more, some less; but it's generally understood that if you stick with something new for a period of time it will become routine. This is good and bad. Good if you are consciously incorporating new healthy things into your life. Bad if you are unconsciously on the gravy train as so many people are.

I try to have at least one juice per day for the nutrients. I insisted on living where I work to reduce wasted commuting time which increased my free time. I then devoted that time to increasing my quality of life. This allowed me to go home every day from the office and have my juice at lunch. This is but one external part of my life that needed to change to "make" free time. So often, the reason I have heard for not doing something, a nice way of saying procrastination, is time. In every moment, we get to choose what we are spending our energy on. And just because you are sitting in traffic or worse, inching along, it doesn't mean that you can't use that time for your goals. Listen to audio books, try soothing music or mindfulness during the periods of perceived wasted time. I blast Frank Sinatra with the windows down in my car and try to make everyone else around me laugh. Make your chosen activities a part of your subconscious, not unconscious, routine and remain conscious when you do it. In other words, as Davidji is fond of saying when describing how to incorporate meditation into your routine: wake up or Rise, then Pee and then Meditate. RPM. You don't have to think about it, simply make it what you do.

Examine your routines—What are you spending your free time on? Do you have free time? Do you have wasted time? Taking my cue from a video game of all places, I started by dividing my time logically into chunks. So much time for work, so much allocated for sleep, relationships, eating, bathing etc. After I divided my day into neat little categories, I started taking a long hard look at what and how I performed whatever I was trying to accomplish during that time slot.

This worked in that it allowed me to really look at how I was living and what my habits were, both good and bad. What I realized was that I had plenty of free time that I had filled up with things, that I thought, were making me happy. In reality, they were actually just escape mechanisms; something to keep my mind occupied as I just couldn't sit silent and still without my mind fixating on something at work or some other stressful situation in life. Our brains are addicted to stimulus and if you're not present and aware, they will get processor time of your consciousness.

Okay, truth time; in my video game mind (I have been playing since the Atari 2600) I liken the concept of balance to the video game "The Sims". In that game, you manage an online avatar as they go through life. You must create and maintain friendly relationships, provide fun through entertainment for you and your friends and of course, you need to perform the basics like sleeping and cooking all the while balancing a career to pay for it all. That game should have been called life. It is for that very reason that I never like the series; it was too real. It felt like life and I was horrible at it. I could never strike the right balance and it would leave my avatar fuming and raging mad.

When I did this exercise, my little routine chart looked something like this:

Food—Every morning was jump started with a vat of coffee; two mugs before leaving home, another when I got to the office. We had a cafeteria in the office so breakfast was bacon and eggs or oatmeal every morning with the coffee. Lunch was whatever was being served in the cafeteria that looked good enough to eat. Dinner was largely a source of protein and some kind of starch; my version of healthy eating at the time. Desert was around 10 PM and could vary from a bag of chips to a bowl of ice cream.

Sleep—Sleep came to me after I had engorged myself into a carbohydrate induced coma most evenings and even then, I would need the TV on to keep my mind from running rampant on me. On average I would get six to eight hours of sleep and feel as if I needed more. I would often let my "entertainment" encroach into this time slot as work often encroached into my entertainment slots.

Relationships—N/A

Eating Habits—I have no dining room table because when I did, I would never use it. I always ate in front of the TV; bad mistake to eat in front of the TV, especially in the unconscious mental state I was in. I would sit down with an entire plate of food and consume the entire plate in less than 15 minutes, all the while not having a clue what I was eating, tasting or watching on TV; as it was just the noise that was necessary to conceal the turmoil in my mind. The end result was that I couldn't hear my body protesting what I was doing to it by eating what I was, and to make matters worse, because I wasn't recognizing that I was eating, even after I had eaten the entire plate of food I still wasn't satisfied. No longer hungry but still wanting to eat.

These are some of the routines I would list on that chart now:

Yoga—Mind body and spirit is what yoga is all about and why it attracted me to it. If balance is my goal, what better activity could I perform? I originally purchased a Yoga DVD to start with, but I soon realized that it only focused on the body, so I expanded my research and practice. I read book after book having not realized just how many different types and styles of yoga there were. I also started realizing that moving slowly, focusing breath and meditating while performing the Yoga was the best way for me to experience it. Yoga is a daily experience for me now. I don't mean just a nice long full session of power yoga, but smaller, multiple times per day events; even if it's simply at the grocery checkout line, standing on one foot.

Walking—I love walking. This is about the only exercise I'm willing to do anymore. I can find a place to walk with Java, my dog, anywhere. I submerse myself into the act of standing fully erect with good posture, placing every step on the ground in exactly the way I wanted to, following my breath, in through the nose expanding the belly first and then up into the chest; exhaling through the nose or mouth depending on how well I'm controlling my exertion. I play with this as I walk, seeing how fast I can walk without needing more oxygen etc. My point is, I get into it with my entire being. It's action meditation or movement meditation.

I'll let you in on a little secret too; remember I used to walk through the Pine Barrens as a teenager? Well, in my twenties, just out of the service and starting my career I lived in an upscale, downtown neighborhood. And assuming I wasn't hung over, and the weather was decent, I used to put on my MP3 player and walk the streets with an attitude or rhythm in the early morning like John Travolta; I have been doing that a lot again lately. There is a dance in my step. Walking is a lot like dancing; the way I walk anyway. It's fast and choreographed to what is playing in my ears, the surroundings I find myself in and the dog who's enjoying it with me. Every step has meaning and purpose. Breathing to fuel the action, fluidity to step accurately and soundly, upper body movements for momentum...

It's action meditation; a gentle grin on my lips, mouth-closed breathing through both nostrils with belly / chest breaths, step by step feeling each section of my body work as I focus on my posture; an occasional attentive adjustment while I remain present to enjoy the world and my dog. I add speed for a challenge and if you focus on walking from the waist down, you can really get moving fast. I get all sorts of looks while I do it but it only makes my smile broader when I discard those thoughts and feel the energy flow. Action meditation; It's all about how you see the world.

Fasting—On a whim, while trying to figure out how to kick start this effort, I decided to take a four day weekend and "clean my system out". I did that by fasting; my version of it anyway. My goal was to see how little I could eat without falling out. Four days isn't enough time to make me fall out, so I added nonstop yoga and meditation into the mix. Be careful and consult a doctor. I already knew how far I could go and I reduced any effort further, whenever I would experiment with a new idea; just in case. This isn't a contest, there is no competition. Speed will actually slow your progress. Space is what you need to create, not speed; you can think of space within an activity as a quiet pause.

Four days of this:

Morning meditation at sunrise with coffee followed by a vigorous walk with the dog. Yoga to stretch out, reading to calm down. Eating consisted of green tea or when really hungry, maybe an orange or a cup of strong coffee. A handful of almonds or natural granola goes a long way as well. Reading after lunch followed by more yoga and an evening walk at dusk. A light meal of some pistachio nuts or almonds and more green tea or water, and if you want something sweet, try some chocolate covered cranberries; just a few. I would then read more or something else relaxing before turning in for the night. Of course, to do this, you need to be at a place where you can spend uninterrupted time, and you need to be relaxed enough to make it work; like on a retreat with Cannabis. How many of us can go to a retreat? Instead, I decided to create a condensed version at home on the weekends. It's a commitment, I understand, but don't fret; meditation is a process that doesn't need to be hastened or cleansed so I'm not recommending you do this. I just happened to feel the need to do it and so I listened to my body and it worked for me.

Seeing as we seem to be a pill popping society let me relate it to you this way. Meditation is like an allergy pill, it needs to build up in your system. The more you meditate, the easier, and more fulfilling it becomes. That first Tuesday morning, after that first long weekend of fasting and meditating, when I went back to work I didn't really feel great but I was much calmer; for a day. I had enough clarity that day however to buy a juicer!

Change my surroundings—Sometimes, you simply must take action that changes your life, if you want to change your life. Sounds stupid but how many people procrastinate? Why? How many talk about change? I clarified one of my biggest fears during a powerful meditative session; money. Here's another point where I will differ with the "normal" world; money is meaningless.

Yes, we have structured our society in such a way where it is required for basic living to have manmade objects (paper money and coins) associated with value so that we can barter something in return for other manmade objects (necessary goods and services) to live. We have thereby created an economy that keeps everyone occupied making money. But, that's all money is, and it's all it's needed for. Everything else is abundance; which is okay too, as long as it too, is balanced with service to humankind. But after you have your basic needs met, and if you agree that everything else is wonderful abundance that can be enjoyed and shared, then why however, do some still seek to amass money? For the sake of trying to have power over others? Could it be viewed as a scorecard of sorts by some? I have personally observed how some are willing to treat others for the sake of personal monetary gain, and I take care to never find myself capable of doing the same. The change I decided to make was to try and change the world; one person at a time. Essentially, I have retired from the rat race; to live a more **Self** centered life while I still can. This has been a wonderful and frightening experience that will not be available to most I completely understand. If you are worrying over a given topic that is making you procrastinate however, ask your Self why. Get to the root cause and understand it. View the answer with a child's innocence and see it for what it is. You'll be amazed at how that changes your perception.

Meditation is not an event but rather a way to walk this earth. It helps if you start from a place of ignorance. I mean it; by starting this myself and only focusing on what is, I was able to look at each moment objectively, I kept asking why to the thoughts that would come into my head while trying to identify their root cause and corresponding emotions. Over and over, every weekend I could devote to it, I would follow roughly the same routine and break down the barriers of my thinking. These are also sometimes referred to as structures.

Meditation is a way to walk this earth objectively and blissfully. I choose my words carefully because I mean to say that I literally now view my walking through a grocery store as a meditation practice.

'Deep breath, am I present or was I still thinking of what to buy inside, or where I was parking, or that jerk at the traffic light?' No judging!

Grocery shopping while being present is fun and great practice for living with compassion, joy and peace which is what this is all about right? "Excuse me" you hear yourself say to another in the store. Now you look around and you are suddenly, if only briefly, aware. That's the moment to step into. That's presence. You were so focused on your perceived life, grocery shopping, that you were actually on autopilot and not aware of the other life around you; you were being managed by your unconscious mind. Then, when you bumped into another human being, shared some atoms somehow, rubbed energy fields maybe who knows, but you snapped back into awareness of your surroundings, thoughts and emotions. Step into it; in military parlance, lean into it. That's present awareness. Hold that level of awareness.

Nature has the same impact on me with one small caveat; nature scales.

If I were around too many people, I used to have a tendency to withdraw inside. I once thought this was fear, and I suppose somehow at some level it was, but I also think its somehow sensory overload, and I believe that's what I'm afraid of. Too many people with minds that are unconsciously chattering away maybe? Nature, however, scales. Walking through the Pine Barrens was a very powerful but calm experience. A shopping mall was a nervous nightmare for me as it was for my mother. I feel more at peace alone in the woods amongst the wildlife than I do in a shopping mall?

Oh boy, down the rabbit hole on that one for a four day weekend and I came to the conclusion that we *must* project our thoughts to one another. If I apply the same logic of starting from peaceful ignorance, I can't deny that the most logical explanation is that what we think, good and bad, actually reflects to what's around us; including each other, and I am apparently a walking antenna! Are we diagnosing that as a disorder instead of recognizing it as evolution? Seriously?

POINTERS

Stop looking at last minute changes as a bad thing. Snap decisions aren't bad either, just insert a pause at the moment of the snap decision or change. Are you aware? Does this thought of decisive action or change bring you and those around you Joy? Why? Feel the emotion. Why that emotion? Is this a pointer? This moment, am I having this thought from a child's like innocent place of peace? If I took action from that decisive thought, what would the goal of that action be? Why? If you can't insert that pause then you are not present.

This observation can be performed in real time but requires strong presence in the moment. I have found that by slowing down and creating pauses, or space, I can function like this, but multitasking still took away from that space. I think this is the trap I was in; not being able to function as I wanted to, I was forced to fall back on my conditioning. What forced the multitasking? What forces us to be harried and rushed all the time? Our persona is the real answer but most of us will blame the office or school or family or some other external entity.

All of the years of conditioning we placed upon ourselves to meet this or that, to achieve, grow, expand; increase shareholder value. All of those events shaped how we think about everything, and that creates reactions or conditional responses. We have conditioned ourselves to dis-ease in many cases. I felt it; and when I did I took responsibility for my **Self** and set out to reverse it quick. In hindsight, there were many much smaller and simpler pointers than a heart attack that I could have paid attention to; if I were only present enough to observe and comprehend them.

Walking the planet in present awareness is my personal and spiritual goal so I can truly live this gift of life. I also feel the need to shout my realizations at the top of my lungs to everyone I meet, but I prefer to not be imprisoned. That's why I want to write about what I've now come to realize. There's a lot of *me* in this paragraph; meaning to be careful not to identify with the thoughts we have of even our own goals and aspirations. Just have them and let it go. Focus back to the present moment, just like meditation. Don't try and plan it out or worry about progress. State your intent and send it out with love and trust. When you have a thought but it's fleeting, something inside you says, whoa, wait, what? Then, your mind starts its analysis. If done consciously from a place of innocent peace and mindfulness, this works to understand your emotions and break down those barriers or conditions; if performed unconsciously however, you may end up identifying with either the thoughts or emotions and all the baggage that comes with them. Now, you are no longer present.

Love and trust was nowhere in me that I could find before I started meditating and yet, love is truly so abundant that it's really hard not to be overwhelmed by it; once you remove the conditions or barriers you have to seeing it. Trust isn't earned however; and it took me quite a long time to come to terms with that one. As a matter of fact, I'm sure I'm still not there. If we project trust, we get trust back. If we don't project trust, we won't get it back; is what I'm down that rabbit-hole with at the moment. Trust is what it takes to be able to let the thoughts that don't serve you go, however. I have learned to not chase my thoughts in that way but I had to trust that extinct first, and I only realized it working after a really good yoga session. I had just sat down to recuperate from my pretzel twisting and an answer to the question I posed to my Self prior to Yoga, clearly and concisely, just popped into my head. It was an "Ah Ha" moment of clarity.

Whenever I realize that I am caught up in thought and emotion rather than being present, I create a mental version of the clapper in my mind's eye. (I can't believe I'm telling you this) Okay, so I consciously tell my mind "Brain Off" and I swear it works for me every time. I, the conscious one, get to decide what my brain is allowed to spend "processor time" on, and I'm peacefully fine with the processor sitting idle at less than one percent utilization. The trick is that I have to observe myself in this state of unconsciousness to be able to snap out of it. This is where pointers help.

There are all sorts of pointers. I view life as a meditation, and the focus of the meditation is to remain present. When we enter into *any* state of suffering, pain or unhappiness, we have lost presence in some way, and once you realize that, your only goal is to get back to the present moment or awareness. In this way, pointers help you to accomplish that.

My cat Tofu loves to sit on my lap while I'm typing at the keyboard. He really prefers me to give him my full attention and a good ear scratching while he sits there; but we've worked out a compromise that suits the both of us. This wonderful life force has been known to jab me with his razor like claws and snap me out of my minds torment over whatever my mind got some processor time on without my permission (unconscious mind). After I noticed it and laughed it off, it happened again. Then again. Now I consider him a part of my growth because of his pointers.

That's a rather simple but profound lesson to be learned. It's wise to walk this planet with no judgment of mind; take every moment for what it is, and use it for right action. Now that mindfulness is becoming more of my normal state, I'm starting to realize the benefits, and I see more and more of these pointers every day. A smile is on my lips more often than not. My gaze has softened a bit. One recent pointer that helped me come to this realization was after I described how I like to have my clothes, including jeans, pressed before wearing them in public. The duffel bag drag is what we called it in the Army when someone wore clothes full of wrinkles. I realized that I was worrying and stressing myself over something as stupid as this when a close friend of mine told me she felt sorry for me.

Really? Why? Because I was so conditioned that just to experience the simple joy of being amongst other humans in a casual atmosphere, I had these rigid rules that only existed in my head for how the moment should be. Then it clicked just like everyone says it does; these rules were in fact limiting my peace and enjoyment of the moment. They had to go. This is how you break down the barriers that create conditional suffering.

I now know that I didn't have a heart attack. It was a panic attack. It was my <u>Self</u> alerting my body to the changes it wanted to make. I didn't realize it at the time of course and it took a bit of time for my machismo to get comfortable with that fact. There was one other doctor, a few years before this event, who woke me up a bit by telling me I needed to love myself more; an odd comment that stuck. There have been other hints and clues that people in this world who have a genuine compassion for others had mentioned to me in the past. They are all wise pointers but only if the person receiving the information is open enough to receive it.

"We do it to ourselves", was another pointer from a person of authority in response to my complaining about chaotic operations at the office. The point I missed at the time of course, was that the chaos was only in my head. It was only real because I perceived it to be real. If I would have taken a step back, taken a deep breath and given the situation a bit of space, I could have realized the moment for what it was, accept it peacefully or at least acknowledge that it is this way for the moment, and then, drop it. If it's wrong and you know it is, ask yourself why? Keep asking why until your inner voice leaves you with no doubt. Now take action to correct it. That's what I call right action.

But how does one go about finding mental tranquility, spiritual awareness and live in peace and loving happiness, all the while holding a day job, in a world full unconscious people, demanding instant gratification and doing more with less work ethics? Maybe I'll be able to put that into a book one day. As for now however, and for the first time in my life, my chosen path was internal. I call it internal because the bulk of what needed to change was within me, not without. I had built structure upon structure by which everything I do and say could be regulated to ensure that what I presented to the world was exactly as it should be to meet my ideals, regardless of what the moment called for. Through meditation, all kinds of meditation, by letting go of personal judgments and trying meditation without any preconceived ideas, I heard myself again. Through dedication and exploration I pushed it. Through Cannabis, I energized it. This is the basics for finding mental tranquility and peace; according to my beliefs.

Balance in all things I knew was the answer. Balance; but how to achieve that? I had some pointers from close friends and colleagues that helped point me in the right direction, but because I'm so thick headed, I didn't know what they were talking about until I had learned it the hard way and then only realized it in reflection. I wrote this book in my usual blunt style so as to penetrate the like-minded thick headed people of this world who often need something to slap them in the face before they recognize it.

Let's get real. I gave myself permission to stop trying to fit in to the mold and simply live the way I want to. I decided to get real and retire from the rat race, move west and immerse myself in humanity now; instead of waiting until I am diseased by the "norm". I wanted to try and live anew, with my new found sanity and knowledge of self so I planned, "The Great Escape"

EPILOGUE: THE GREAT ESCAPE–TRAVELLING ACROSS AMERICA.

Finally, a nice scenic place to get out of the car with the dog and meditate on my yoga mat for a while. It was a beautiful rest area on I-84 in Oregon; not far from Portland. We had started the day at sunrise; in Salt Lake City, UT. Although we drove across country with no planning, just letting our nose point the way, we planned this one part of our trip just so we could drive this last stretch in daylight. This stretch of road is what my memory of the west has been for twenty years; a deep ravine with a river at the bottom as you drive the snake of an interstate alongside. This was the northwest! I had hoped to find such a restful place with easy access and start to enjoy my new beginning and here it was; and it didn't disappoint.

After a wonderful 30 minutes or so of peaceful meditation, off of a trail from a rest area in the ravine, Java, my ever present mini American Shepherd and I started back to the car and met a very friendly gentleman with his dog. We let the two dogs play for a while as we engaged in light conversation;

What kind of dog? How old? Where you headed? What do you do? When we thought the dogs had enough, we said our goodbyes and on the way back to the car I thought, "Huh, west coast is friendly".

As I got back to my car, a woman sitting on a stone wall in front of my car commented on my dog (people love my dog and think she was born so well trained; they hardly ever notice me other than being her "handler") and again in the spirit of getting into the west coast mindset, I stopped to chat it up a bit.

Thirty seconds later, Gertrude (not her real name) had told me, in tears, that she was a laid off software developer but was thinking of getting into Cyber Security. In my new way of seeing the world, I thought I could help Gertrude; seeing as I had just left a 20 year career in Technology, specifically in Cyber Security for the last few. It truly was the very last topic I would have wanted to discuss, but it was a subject I knew well, so I thought I could dispense my sage wisdom with an honest dose of reality and get back to my scenic journey west.

Then Hank walked over (real name), and Gertrude introduced him as her husband; and that was my last chance to speak;

"Nice to meet you"

"Get 'em Hotchkiss; how about a fast ride to San Francisco in that car of yours?"

"Huh, er wha.."

"He's from Maryland hunny"

"Oh, we protested last week, how much did you see?"

"I'm sorry?"

"We protested last week in Portland, how much did you see in DC?"

"I'm sorry I don't watch the news.."

"You're not missing anything"

"Heh, yeah…"

"How much did you see?"

"What were you protesting?"

"Monsanto, man"

"What did Monsanto do?"

"Monsanto man, we protested last week and let me tell you about some conspiracy that….. "

At that point I decided to use my dog to my advantage and as an excuse. I literally started bowing and pointing to my dog as if to say "Oh dear wonderful people, all wrapped up tight in your egoic existence, if I don't get my dog back into this car and get to driving west, she will die a painful death one thousand times over." I sped off thinking; left coast nuttiness, alive and well. Then I reminded myself not to judge and I immediately knew this was going to be a challenging time; and then I got giddy in anticipation.

Travelling across America is a great experience that far too many people overlook. Let me tell you briefly about this journey.

"You're going to drive there?"

If I had a dollar for every time I heard that when I was discussing my "Great Escape", I certainly wouldn't need for money again. But let's not get ahead of ourselves, you see, this "Great Escape" was me leaving the funny farm, or as most "normal" people call it, Corporate America. I had spent 20 years in Information Technology in various positions. I was negative and miserable despite making a good living and having pretty good job stability; job stability that is, until you get into your fifties and corporate America kicks you to the curb.

Thanks for your 30 years of service Gertrude, but your programming skills aren't needed anymore and instead of mentoring you or teaching you new skills, we decided that your health care is costing us too much money; and you know, shareholder value (code language for executive bonus structure) is our number one priority.

I was 42 and decided to get the jump on retirement instead of waiting around to be a burden to shareholder value; I wanted to live a little for a change, and I had always wanted to live out west. Don't ask me that, I don't know where. I fell in love with New Mexico, Montana, Colorado, Nebraska, Wyoming, Oregon, Idaho and Washington. I like big open space where you can see the curvature of the earth with a crystal clear blue sky and little humidity because you're so high in elevation. Now, punctuate that vision with a snow capped mountain. That's where I want to live; that's my escape. Where is that?

Yes, I drove across the country. Maybe I'm getting old but I remember camping as great fun; travel trailers, singing in the car, CB radio. I remember when truck drivers had respect on the road because it was deserved; same with public safety officials. Take a train if you don't want to drive or take a bus, but don't fly over those states. Get out, mingle and share a few atoms. There are lots of fantastic people, places and things of nature to be celebrated; not overlooked. Yes, driving across country is great fun and educational. It's a pleasure to be able to do it and I liken it to a vacation that we ALL richly deserve; one of discovering ourselves.

When I decided to make my dream of living out west a reality, I set my life up in such a way as to be able to take advantage of whatever opportunities came my way that would help me realize that dream. I didn't set out to *make* the opportunities present themselves however until one day, when I suddenly realized that twenty years had gone by since I started my technology career; I resigned. That was a pointer I decided to listen to.

Amassing money can be dangerously addictive and while I completely understand the incredible amount of money involved with putting kids through college, there are plenty who are past that point and yet they keep going and going like the energizer bunny, until they suffer from a chronic disease that overwhelms their body. Not me; I'd like to live a little before my body dies thanks.

My new career is to immerse myself in humanity, help where I can and write about it. Halfway houses, public nursing homes, mental institutions are all in the works hopefully with my wonderful American Shepherd "Java" as a therapy dog. So, my plan was simple really; drive around the states I felt drawn to, until I found a place that spoke to me. I've never seen the movie Thelma and Louise but that was what I called it. I simply loaded the essentials into the car for a week long journey.

I had a hard criterion to meet too. The location had to have very reliable Internet access. If I were going to immerse myself in humanity, I couldn't isolate myself on a mountain top either; there had to be humanity around for the immersion. Add to that, I wanted it cheap so I wouldn't have as many worries about paying the bills etc. I was also determined not to pre-judge anywhere until I saw it, and promised to venture off the beaten path along the way looking for places I didn't think of before.

It was a great ride. It was brutal.

There are two seasons on the US Interstate system in America; winter and construction. Now, I love to drive, and I usually *really* drive, but the car was loaded down with the essentials necessary for me, my cat and my dog to live for a few days and the essentials we would initially need in any new place we may find. As an aside, in a very typical male fashion, I realized after I unpacked the car, my view of essentials is a bit askew. For example, I brought my primary desktop computer powerhouse, complete with three twenty something inch widescreen monitors and its corresponding audio and video recording systems with me in the car; the tools of my new trade. But I didn't bring a spoon, or a jacket, or even long pants. I figured there will always be Walmart's. I brought a small digital camera for taking quick shots, but the charger was buried somewhere that I had no chance of finding because my hastily created luggage was a roll of hefty bags. I was felling, and acting, like the last twenty years didn't happen and I was twenty two instead of forty two and starting all over again.

Needless to say, my car was loaded down with 'useless at the time' items. It was very hot and humid when I left Maryland and although I knew the humidity would be less elsewhere, I figured its summertime, it can't get *that* cold; and again, anything I may need is just a Walmart away. I didn't account for the fact that stores only carry seasonal items anymore. Not even as much as a light jacket or a hoodie; in five different super Walmart's that I stopped in. It's quite cold, even during the day in the summer, out west, I now admit. During this brief tour of America, I saw truck stops, Walmart's and motels much more frequently than I did peaceful meditative places and it occurred to me that despite the enormous "bail-out" packages from the 2008 financial crisis, the interstate system is in horrible shape! How could none of that money have gone to employing people to actually work on repairing or upgrading a critical part of our infrastructure?

Here's an economical tip when "hoofing it" across country in your "four wheeler". Don't overlook the idea of sleeping in your car in rest areas or at truck / travel stops while travelling; they really are for everyone—trucks, motor homes and cars. Loves is the name of a chain I have a lot of respect for and after you uncramp your back from trying to get at least a few hours of shut eye inside your car, you can go inside the store and enjoy a nice clean hot shower and a steaming cup of coffee for ten dollars. Much cheaper than a motel and, at least you know who's been sleeping in your car at night. Don't be bashful; carry your toilet bag and clean clothes to the counter. That's all you need to do.

Truck drivers never liked the mixing of the general public in "their" truck stops largely because of the way the general public looked at the way some of the drivers live! This was their space and they didn't like being ridiculed; and they shouldn't be. As a matter of fact, try joining them. Think about the last time you were driving at night on the interstate, maybe you didn't know the area and nobody else was around; except a truck driver. Did you get a feeling of comfort knowing that, if nothing else, there was another human around? Now, what if it's really late, you're very tired, it's hilly terrain with many curves. You would pull over, but you are literally on a roller coaster of a road and there's nowhere to stop. You can drive as fast as 70 mph, but a truck can only go as fast as 60 mph legally. You don't care and slow down anyway to follow that truck. Why? Always ask why. Because you are trusting that professional driver with your life. You are trusting him or, very commonly her, to guide you through this hellava road until you can get to a safe place to stop. Then when you do, you cast that driver a silent thank you as you go to sleep.

That's the very same person you could be turning your nose up at, the next morning getting coffee, as your thoughts automatically "judge" that truck driver for some reason or another. Think about what it takes for them to do their job. This is how they live and it's a very feasible way to travel as well. Remember, no judging. Yes, travelling across country is much more luxurious in a coach or motorhome, don't get me wrong, but a decent car, or eighteen wheeler will work as well. Be non-judgmental and accepting, we are all the same; human. Working the interstate system, as I refer to it as, was a common approach that I took throughout this trip; I'm retired from the rat race now after all and I need to be frugal.

We spent a night in Utah in anticipation of a wonderful drive through Oregon on Interstate 84 during the next day. By then, we had just met Gertrude and Hank. Oregon would have had me, lock stock and barrel except for one small fact; marijuana is legal to consume in Washington; and any state that sees the benefits of cannabis enough to legalize its use must be full of relaxed and groovy people right? I pressed on toward Seattle.

Maybe driving all day made me a bit on edge, but my first impression of Monday evening rush hour traffic around the I5 corridor north of Portland was, lawlessness on the roads. My impression of the atmosphere in Washington State in general, is one of personal freedom and tolerance. We drove the I5 to Seattle, then went east to Spokane, and then Southwest until we hit Portland again over the next couple of days to get an updated feel for the state, as it had been twenty years since I had last been to Washington. When all was said and done, we picked Tacoma Washington as our final destination, as it met all the criteria; including the snowcapped mountain.

We are all humans and we are all interconnected as one. As soon as we realize that, the world will be much better off I suspect, so Java and I will do what we can, when we can, to help that realization come to the masses; starting right here in Tacoma. We'll blog about it at lifetheblog.com and attempt to help raise awareness to issues that need the attention for the betterment of humanity through the written word.

It isn't easy trying to live the way you want to live. Honestly, it's much easier to go along and get along; but if we are to evolve as a species, if we are to truly overcome our differences for the sake of humanity, then perhaps we should all become less conditioned, less unconscious and more compassionately aware. That's easy to say when nothing is at risk. It's easy to follow principals when there are nor repercussions. I challenge everyone to live how they believe every moment of their existence.

If you just thought to yourself "That's it"? "This is the end of the book"? Then perhaps I can sum the entire book up into one clear sentence. Make the time to sit quietly by yourself, every day, and trust your inner being to guide you the rest of the way. That's all I really needed to put into the book…. but who would buy it then?

I started this search for balance by standing on one foot. I'm still standing. Namaste

www.ingramcontent.com/pod-product-compliance
Lightning Source LLC
Chambersburg PA
CBHW020338290526
45785CB00005B/2081